Type 2 Diabetes:

The Basics and Overall Management

Richard Westman

TABLE OF CONTENTS

INTRODUCTION 1

OVERVIEW 3

SYMPTOMS OF TYPE 2 DIABETES.. 18

DIET FOR TYPE 2 DIABETES 20

TREATMENT FOR TYPE 2 DIABETES.. 32

CAUSES OF TYPE 2 DIABETES 34

MEDICATIONS FOR TYPE 2 DIABETES... 37

TYPE 2 DIABETES IN CHILDREN 43

RISK FACTORS FOR TYPE 2 DIABETES 45

TIPS FOR HOW TO PREVENT TYPE 2 DIABETES 48

PREVENTING DIABETES PROBLEMS 52

RECEIVING A TYPE 2 DIABETES DIAGNOSIS 55

COMPLICATIONS ASSOCIATED WITH TYPE 2 DIABETES........... 64

MANAGING TYPE 2 DIABETES 66

STEPS TO FIGHT DIABETES WITHOUT MEDICATION 76

THE SAFEST FIRST-LINE THERAPY FOR TYPE 2 DIABETES..... 78

EXERCISE TIPS FOR TYPE 2 DIABETES....................................... 81

THE IMPORTANCE OF EXERCISE IN FIGHTING TYPE 2
DIABETES.. 84

HOW TO FIGHT DIABETES EFFECTIVELY 86

MASSAGE THERAPY FOR DIABETES 88

INTRODUCTION

Diabetes is a disease in which the glucose in the blood is higher than normal. High blood glucose is called hyperglycemia.

Glucose is a type of sugar that comes from foods containing carbohydrates and is found in everyone's blood. Glucose is transported through the blood to all tissues and organs to be used for energy.

Definition of diabetes: Blood glucose should not be too low (hypoglycemia) or too high (hyperglycemia). The body usually keeps blood glucose within a certain range. When blood glucose begins to rise above normal, it either enters cells to be used for energy, or it is stored. If it is stored for future use, it will be converted to glycogen or fat. Glycogen is a "quick fuel"that is found in muscle and the liver.

The body is normally able to control blood glucose levels using of a hormone called insulin. Insulin is released by the pancreas in response to increased levels of glucose in the blood. Insulin, blood glucose and the cell's receptor all work together to move the glucose into the cell.

With diabetes, however, the body has trouble making or using insulin. For this reason, blood glucose levels rise and hyperglycemia occurs.

To imagine how glucose, insulin, and cell receptors work, think of your car. To park in your garage, you need a garage door and a garage door opener. Glucose is like your car, the cell receptor is like the garage door, and the insulin is like the opener.

If your body does not make enough insulin or if it does not work properly, glucose cannot get into your cells. Instead, glucose stays in your blood causing high blood glucose, or hyperglycemia. People with hyperglycemia have diabetes.

OVERVIEW

Diabetes is a disease in which blood glucose levels are above normal. Most of the food we eat is turned into glucose, or sugar, for our bodies to use for energy. The pancreas, an organ that lies near the stomach, makes a hormone called insulin to help glucose get into the cells of our bodies. When you have diabetes, your body either doesn't make enough insulin or can't use its own insulin as well as it should. This causes sugar to build up in your blood.

Diabetes can cause serious health complications including heart disease, blindness, kidney failure, and lower-extremity amputations. Diabetes is the seventh leading cause of death in the United States.

Carbohydrates, Proteins, and Fats all Contain Calories

To understand and manage diabetes well, you must know what happens to food when you eat. Food is made of

- Carbohydrates

- Proteins

- Fats

- Vitamins

- Minerals

- Water

Carbohydrates, proteins, and fats all contain calories, and can all be used for energy. Carbohydrates are mostly in foods in the starchy foods groups, but also in vegetables, fruits, dairy foods, and sugars. The primary sources of protein are meats and dairy products. Fat can be found in dairy and meats. Fat can also be added to food, such as salad dressing or margarine. Fat can also be added when food is made, such as chips, cookies, or pizza.

Too many calories can cause weight gain. Weight gain usually also results in higher blood glucose levels because the body becomes less sensitive to insulin.

Vitamins, minerals, and water do not contain calories, cannot be used for energy, and do not affect blood glucose.

How does food turn into glucose?

When we eat, carbohydrates, proteins, and fats are digested and broken into smaller parts. Once broken down, these parts will affect blood glucose differently depending on how they are absorbed and how the body uses them.

Almost all the carbohydrates eaten will be converted into glucose in the body. The only carbohydrates not changed to glucose are those that cannot be digested, like fiber.

Protein and fat are not directly converted to glucose when digested. The effect on blood glucose is not as direct as eating carbohydrate. Eating too much protein and fat can lead to eating too many calories. Too many calories can make the cell insensitive to insulin. If the cell is insensitive to insulin, blood glucose can rise. So the amount of food that's eaten can affect blood glucose – too much can lead to weight gain, insulin resistance, and higher blood glucose levels. Carbohydrates affect blood glucose, because carbohydrates are digested and broken into smaller parts that are primarily glucose units.

Is Glucose Bad for People with Diabetes?

No, glucose is not bad for people with diabetes. Everyone, including people with diabetes, needs glucose for energy. We need energy to play, exercise, and work, but we also need it for everyday body functions, like breathing, digesting, and making blood cells. Most of the glucose in our body comes from eating carbohydrates.

Everyone needs glucose for energy

People without diabetes are able to keep their blood glucose levels in a normal range regardless of the amount they eat. For people with diabetes, it is harder to keep blood glucose in a normal range. For this reason, people with diabetes need to balance the amount of food that they eat (especially food that contains carbohydrates) with their medication and activity level.

Why do Some People have High Blood Glucose Levels?

Mainly foods containing carbohydrates are broken down into glucose and used for energy. Once food is broken down into glucose, it enters the blood and is carried to all the cells of the body. However, in order for glucose to enter the cell, a special helper and cell receptor are needed. The helper that glucose needs to enter the cell is called insulin. Insulin is a hormone made by the pancreas. Cell receptors are like doorways into a cell. A cell can have many receptors.

How glucose and insulin normally work?

If your body does not make enough insulin or if the insulin or the cell receptors do not work the way they should, glucose cannot get into your cells. Instead, glucose stays in your blood causing hyperglycemia. A complete lack of insulin results in type 1 diabetes. Insulin or cell receptors that do not work properly result in type 2 diabetes.

Are there Different Types of Diabetes?

Diabetes is not one single condition. Researchers are discovering many different reasons for diabetes to develop in one person rather than another. Some of these newer types of diabetes include maturity onset of the young diabetes, latent autoimmune diabetes, and chemically or surgically induced diabetes.

In all types of diabetes, blood glucose is higher than it should be. It is the reason that it is high that makes the types of diabetes different. Generally, however, there are three main types of diabetes:

- type 1 diabetes

- type 2 diabetes

- gestational diabetes

TYPE 1 DIABETES

Glucose can't get into the cell, because no insulin is produced by the body.

Type 1 diabetes can occur at any age, but is most often diagnosed early in life. Type 1 diabetes is called an autoimmune disease, because the immune system attacks the person's own cells. In this type of diabetes, cells in the pancreas that produce insulin are the target of the body's immune system and are eventually destroyed. For this reason, people with type 1 diabetes produce no insulin so glucose cannot get into the cells.

Symptoms of type 1 diabetes include:

- Weight loss
- Thirst (polydipsia)
- Extreme hunger (polyphagia)
- Excessive urination (polyuria)
- Weakness or tiredness

The symptoms of type 1 diabetes all relate to the high blood glucose levels. The glucose does not keep into the cell so the cell can't do its work. This causes weight loss and tiredness. Because the glucose can't get into the cell, the cell also signals that it needs glucose (food) and extreme hunger results. With the high blood glucose, there is an increased excretion of glucose into the urine. This also pulls more water with the glucose to keep the urine less concentrated. These two things cause increased thirst and increased urination.

TYPE 2 DIABETES

Cell receptors are not working to let insulin-glucose enter the cell.

Type 2 diabetes is the most common form of diabetes. Ninety-five percent of the people who have diabetes have type 2.

Although it was once thought that type 2 diabetes occurred only in adults, it is now known that people can develop type 2 diabetes at any age. With type 2 diabetes, the receptors on the cells become resistant to insulin and therefore cannot let glucose into the cell.

Type 2 diabetes may also result if the body does not make enough insulin. Both problems with the cell receptor or with the amount of insulin produced, lead to high blood glucose levels. Being overweight and inactive increases the chance of developing type 2 diabetes.

Insulin resistance is a condition when normal insulin levels do not result in glucose entry into the cell. Higher than normal insulin levels in the blood occur in insulin resistance.

People who have insulin resistance are usually overweight or obese. They may have a normal blood glucose, be diagnosed as "pre-diabetes," or have type 2 diabetes. People who have a normal blood glucose may have no symptoms of insulin resistance but usually develop pre-diabetes. Those with pre-diabetes usually develop type 2 diabetes. The exception to this progression occurs when overweight or obese people lose weight, eat a healthy diet, and exercise regularly.Not everyone who is obese or overweight will develop insulin resistance, although a lot of people will. Genetics, diet, and activity levels all can play an important role in how well insulin and glucose interact.

Symptoms of type 2 diabetes include:

- Frequent urination (polyuria)

- Thirst (polydipsia)

- Blurred vision

- Unintentional weight gain or weight loss, although little weight change may occur Fatigue

However, many people have no noticeable symptoms. This is because type 2 diabetes develops over a long time, usually several years. With these gradual changes in insulin resistance and glucose tolerance, a person may not notice symptoms as unusual, especially if they are older. For instance, blurry vision that could occur due to damage by high blood glucose to the eye could be mistaken for normal eye changes with aging.

Another possible symptom of type 2 diabetes is slow wound healing. The high blood glucose prevents the normal healing process from occurring, and cuts or scrapes take a very long time to heal. Another possible symptom of type 2 diabetes in women is multiple urinary tract infections. The increased excretion of high levels of glucose also attract yeast, and can cause an infection.

GESTATIONAL DIABETES

Gestational diabetes is a form of diabetes that occurs during pregnancy. When a woman becomes pregnant there are many hormonal changes that take place. These changes, especially in the later stages of pregnancy, can affect the mother's sensitivity to insulin. When the mother becomes resistant to insulin, her cells do not let glucose in and her blood glucose levels rise. When blood glucose levels rise above a certain level, gestational diabetes is diagnosed.

Doctors often check women's blood glucose levels during their pregnancy because high blood glucose levels can cause complications during the pregnancy or after the baby is born. These complications include infants of high birth weight, increased risk of cesarean delivery, infant respiratory distress syndrome, infant hypoglycemia following delivery, and infant jaundice. The presence of fasting hyperglycemia greater than 105mg/dl may be associated with increased risk of fetal malformations and death. Although gestational diabetes usually goes away after the baby's birth, women with this type of diabetes are at high risk for developing type 2 diabetes later in life.

Treatment Goals

There are certain goals set by the American Diabetes Association.

Maintain a near-normal level of blood glucose. This can only be achieved by balancing the amount of food eaten with the amount exercise performed, and the amount of insulin available and effective. The insulin can be either what the body makes (endogenous) or be insulin injections (exogenous).

Oral glucose-lowering medications and physical activity can also help maintain normal glucose levels. Achieve and/or maintain optimal blood lipid levels. Achieve and/or maintain optimal weight.

Prevent and/or treat complications of diabetes, such as retinopathy, kidney disease, neuropathy, and cardiovascular disease. Include healthy eating and maintain pleasure in eating. Be able to plan meals to fit your lifestyle.

Health care providers also recommend achieving normal blood pressure levels as a treatment goal. Goals concerning the treatment of diabetes

Meal Planning

The purpose of meal planning is to help you reach your personal blood glucose or weight goals. These goals should be discussed with your health care provider. How these goals are achieved will be different for everyone. Some may reach their goals by spacing their food intake and limiting portion sizes. Others benefit from a more specific meal plan. Serving sizes are always important when you plan your meals. Day-to-day variation in meals and snacks can lead to uneven glucose pattern.

Blood glucose levels are affected by the timing of meals and snacks Blood glucose levels are affected by the timing of meals and snacks.

Commonly used methods of meal planning include:

- The Plate Method

- MyPlate

- Exchange Lists

- Carbohydrate Counting

The Plate Method: Breakfast, Lunch/Dinner

The plate method is one way that meals can be planned. For breakfast, starch should take up half of the plate, and meat or non-meat protein may take up 1/4 of the plate if desired. In the lunch and dinner plate method, vegetables should take up half of the plate, starch should take up 1/4 of the plate and meat or non-meat protein should take up another 1/4 of the plate. One serving of fruit and a cup of low-fat milk may accompany your meal.

Although the plate method is relatively easy, portion sizes are still critical. The amount of food on your plate should vary according to the number of calories that you need each day. A recommended plate size is about 9 inches across (9 inch diameter). Try measuring your plates!

Starchy foods include: bread, rolls, rice, pasta, potatoes, yams, corn, lima beans, and cereals.

Vegetables include: lettuce, tomatoes, mushrooms, spinach, green beans, and broccoli.

Meat and non-meat protein foods include: chicken, beef, pork, fish, cheese, beans, tofu, and soy products that resemble meat or chicken.

MyPlate

MyPlate is a tool used to show the type and the amount of food that you need daily. Recently modified to take into consideration the new Dietary Guidelines for Americans, the new MyPlate has a plate divided into four sections and a glass for diary.

MyPlate suggests that you:

- Make half your grains whole grains

- Make have your plate fruits and vegetables

- Switch to fat-free or low-fat milk

- Find your balance between food and physical activity

- Choose lower sodium foods

- Drink water instead of sugary drinks

Exchange Lists

There are six different Exchange List groups including the starch groups, the fruit group, the milk group, the non-starchy vegetable group, the meat and meat substitutes group, and the fat group. Each serving of food within an exchange group has about the same amount of carbohydrate, protein, fat, and calories as the other foods in that group. For this reason, foods within an exchange list group can be substituted for each other, but foods on one group list cannot be substituted for foods on another group list. For example, you may substitute eating a small apple for a small orange, because they are both one serving in the fruit group. However, you could not substitute eating a small apple for one slice of bread, because these foods are in different groups.

The amount and type of exchanges recommended each day are based on individual calorie needs, weight goals and the amount of physical activity performed daily

The following are the six groups of the Diabetic

i. Starches List (Includes bread, cereals, grains and starchy vegetables) One exchange from this group has 15 grams of carbohydrates, 3 grams of protein, and 0-1g of fat for a total of 80 calories per serving.

Examples of one serving from this group include 1 slice of bread, 1/3 cup cooked rice, or 1/3 cup cooked pasta.

ii. Fruit List

One exchange from this group has 15 grams of carbohydrate for a total of 60 calories per serving. Foods in the fruit list do not contain any protein or fat. Examples of one serving from this group include 1 small apple, 17 small grapes, or ½ cup of orange juice.

iii. Non-starchy Vegetable List

One exchange from this group has 2 grams of carbohydrates, and 5 grams of protein for a total of 25 calories per serving. Non-starchy vegetables contain no fat. Examples of one serving from this group include 1/2 cup cooked green beans, 1 cup raw lettuce, or 1/2 cup vegetable juice.

iv. Milk List

Milk List Items on the milk list are divided into fat-free/low-fat milk, reduced-fat milk, and whole milk categories.

One fat-free/low-fat milk exchange has 12 grams of carbohydrates, 8 grams of protein, and 0-3g of fat for a total of 90 calories per serving. One reduced-fat milk exchange has 12 grams of carbohydrates, 8 grams of protein, and 5g of fat for a total of 120 calories per serving. One whole milk exchange has 12 grams of carbohydrates, 8 grams of protein, and 8g of fat for a total of 150 calories per serving. Examples of one serving from the fat-free/low-fat milk exchange are 1 cup of non-fat skim or 1% milk, or 2/3 cup (or 6 ounces) of fat-free plain yogurt.

v. Meat and Meat Substitutes ListMeat

Meats are divided into very lean, lean, medium-fat, and high-fat lists based on the amount of fat they contain. High-fat exchanges should be eaten a maximum of three times a week. One very lean meat exchange has 7 grams of protein, and 0-1 gram of fat for a total of 35 calories per serving. Examples of one very lean meat exchange are 1 ounce white meat chicken or turkey with no skin. One lean meat exchange has 7 grams of protein, and 3 grams of fat for a total of 55 calories per serving. Examples of one lean meat exchange are 1 ounce lean beef or lean pork.

One medium-fat meat exchange has 7 grams of protein, and 5 grams of fat for a total of 75 calories per serving. Examples of one medium-fat meat exchange are 1 ounce dark meat chicken with skin, 1 egg, or 1 ounce of fried fish.

One high-fat meat exchange has 7 grams of protein, and 8 grams of fat for a total of 100 calories per serving. Examples of one high-fat meat exchange are 1 ounce pork sausage, 1 ounce American cheese, or 1ounce of a hot dog.

Whereas one exchange from this list only refers to a 1 ounce portion of meat or meat substitute, a serving refers to 2 - 3 ounce portions of the foods in this list. A serving is often used in referring to the foods in this group because most people eat more than one ounce of meat or meat substitutes at a time.

vi. Fat List

Fat List One exchange from this group has 5 grams of fat for a total of 45 calories per serving. Most items in the fat exchange list do not contain protein or carbohydrate.

Examples of one serving from this group include one teaspoon oil, one teaspoon butter, one teaspoon mayonnaise, or one tablespoon salad dressing.

Carbohydrate Counting: The Carbohydrate Counting method is similar to the Exchange List method in that they both use food groups. However, when you use Carbohydrate Counting, you keep track or "count" servings equal to 15 grams or 1 unit of carbohydrate The food groups that have carbohydrate and are counted are:

The Starch and Starchy Vegetables Group

   The Fruit Group

   The Milk Group

One serving from any of these three groups would count as one carbohydrate unit. For example if you ate two pieces of buttered toast and an 8 ounce glass of milk for breakfast, you would count that breakfast as having three carbohydrate units. Carbohydrate Counting differs from the Exchange List in that the amount of protein and fats in foods is not taken into consideration. So the butter on the toast consumed at breakfast would not be counted, because butter is in the fat group and does not contain carbohydrate.

Some examples of one carbohydrate unit would be:

Starch and Starchy Vegetables Group – 1 slice of bread, 1/3 cup of cooked rice or pasta, 1/2 of a small bagel

Milk Group – 1 cup milk, 2/3 cup fat-free-yogurt, 3/4 cup low-fat yogurt

Fruit Group – 1 small piece of fruit, 3/4 cup berries, 1/2 cup apple juice

If you are planning to use the Carbohydrate Counting method, you and your health care provider should decide how many servings of carbohydrate you should consume each day and at each meal for optimal health.

Managing your Diabetes

How does someone with diabetes make sure they get the right amount of glucose, carbohydrates, or energy without their blood glucose getting too high? Remember that the food you eat is the energy that has to be balanced with exercise, which uses energy. The food that is best for someone who has diabetes isn't magic or tasteless or unusual. It is regular food in the right amounts. Managing your diabetes will reduce your risk for complications of diabetes and help you feel better on a daily basis.

The management of diabetes has three parts:

- Making healthy food choices

- Participating in physical activity

- Taking your prescribed medications

One way to see if you are managing your diabetes effectively is to monitor your blood glucose daily. Self-monitoring of blood glucose (SMBG) allows you to check your blood glucose level with a glucose meter and glucose testing strip and see if you are at, above, or below the normal blood glucose range. SMBG makes it easy for you to check your blood glucose wherever you are and whenever it is convenient for you. It is important to check your blood glucose level daily, but ask your doctor how many times a day you should check your blood glucose level for best monitoring.

SYMPTOMS OF TYPE 2 DIABETES

Diabetes is a medical condition in which sugar, or glucose, levels build up in your bloodstream. There's not enough insulin to move the sugar into your cells, which are where the sugar is used for energy. This causes your body to rely on alternative energy sources in your tissues, muscles, and organs.

This is a chain reaction that can cause a variety of symptoms. Type 2 diabetes can develop slowly. The symptoms may be mild and easy to dismiss at first.

The early symptoms may include:

- constant hunger

- ack of energy

- fatigue

- weight loss

- excessive thirst

- frequent urination

- dry mouth

- itchy skin

- blurry vision

As the disease progresses, the symptoms become more severe and potentially dangerous.

If your blood sugar levels have been high for a long time, the symptoms can include:

- yeast infections

- slow-healing cuts or sores

- dark patches on your skin

- foot pain

- feelings of numbness and tingling in your hands/feet, or neuropathy

If you have two or more of these symptoms, you should see your doctor. Without treatment, diabetes can become life-threatening.

Diabetes has a powerful effect on your heart. Women with diabetes are twice as likely to have another heart attack after the first one. They're at quadruple the risk of heart failure when compared to women without diabetes. Diabetes can also lead to complications during pregnancy.

DIET FOR TYPE 2 DIABETES

Diet is an important tool to keep your heart healthy and blood sugar levels within a safe and healthy range. It doesn't have to be complicated or unpleasant. The diet recommended for people with type 2 diabetes is the same diet just about everyone should follow. It boils down to a few key actions:

- Eat meals and snacks on schedule.

- Choose a variety of foods that are high in nutrition and low in empty calories.

- Be careful not to overeat.

- Read food labels closely.

- Foods to choose

- Healthy carbohydrates can provide you with fiber.

The options include:

- Vegetables

- Fruits

- Legumes, such as beans

- Whole grains

Foods with heart-healthy omega-3 fatty acids include:

- Tuna

- Sardines

- Salmon

- Mackerel

- Halibut

- cod

You can get healthy monounsaturated and polyunsaturated fats from a number of foods, including:

- olive oil

- canola oil

- peanut oil

- almonds

- pecans

- walnuts

- avocados

Although these options for fat are good for you, they're high in calories. Moderation is key. When choosing dairy products, choose low-fat options.

There are certain foods that you should limit or avoid entirely. These include:

- foods heavy in saturated fats

- foods heavy in trans fats

- beef

- processed meats

- shellfish

- organ meats, such as beef or liver

- stick margarine

- shortening

- baked goods

- processed snacks

- sugary drinks

- high-fat dairy products

- salty foods

- fried foods

Talk to your doctor about your personal nutrition and calorie goals. Together, you can come up with a diet plan that tastes great and suits your lifestyle needs.

Diabetes Diet, Eating, & Physical Activity

Nutrition and physical activity are important parts of a healthy lifestyle when you have diabetes. Along with other benefits, following a healthy meal plan and being active can help you keep your blood glucose level, also called blood sugar, in your target range. To manage your blood glucose, you need to balance what you eat and drink with physical activity and diabetes medicine if you take any. What you choose to eat, how much you eat, and when you eat are all important in keeping your blood glucose level in the range that your health care team recommends.

Becoming more active and making changes in what you eat and drink can seem challenging at first. You may find it easier to start with small changes and get help from your family, friends, and health care team.

Eating well and being physically active most days of the week can help you keep your blood glucose level, blood pressure, and cholesterol in your target ranges

- lose weight or stay at a healthy weight

- prevent or delay diabetes problems

- feel good and have more energy

What foods can I eat if I have diabetes?

You may worry that having diabetes means going without foods you enjoy. The good news is that you can still eat your favorite foods, but you might need to eat smaller portions or enjoy them less often. Your health care team will help create a diabetes meal plan for you that meets your needs and likes.

The key to eating with diabetes is to eat a variety of healthy foods from all food groups, in the amounts your meal plan outlines.

The food groups are

Vegetables nonstarchy: includes broccoli, carrots, greens, peppers, and tomatoes

starchy: includes potatoes, corn, and green peas

fruits—includes oranges, melon, berries, apples, bananas, and grapes

grains—at least half of your grains for the day should be whole grains includes wheat, rice, oats, cornmeal, barley, and quinoa examples: bread, pasta, cereal, and tortillas

protein:

- lean meat

- chicken or turkey without the skin

- fish

- eggs

- nuts and peanuts

- dried beans and certain peas, such as chickpeas and split peas

   meat substitutes, such as tofudairy—nonfat or low fat milk or lactose-free milk if you have lactose intolerance

- yogurt

- cheese

Eat foods with heart-healthy fats, which mainly come from these foods:

- oils that are liquid at room temperature, such as canola and olive oil

- nuts and seeds

   heart-healthy fish such as salmon, tuna, and mackerel avocado

Use oils when cooking food instead of butter, cream, shortening, lard, or stick margarine.

Photo of avocado, salmon, nuts, seeds, and olive oil. Choose healthy fats, such as from nuts, seeds,

and olive oil.

What foods and drinks should I limit if I have diabetes?

Foods and drinks to limit include: fried foods and other foods high in saturated

- fat and trans fat

- foods high in salt, also called sodium

- sweets, such as baked goods, candy, and ice cream

- beverages with added sugars, such as juice, regular soda, and regular sports or energy drinks

Drink water instead of sweetened beverages. Consider using a sugar substitute in your coffee or tea.

If you drink alcohol, drink moderately—no more than one drink a day if you're a woman or two drinks a day if you're a man. If you use insulin or diabetes medicines that increase the amount of insulin your body makes, alcohol can make your blood glucose level drop too low. This is especially true if you haven't eaten in a while. It's best to eat some food when you drink alcohol.

When should I eat if I have diabetes?

Some people with diabetes need to eat at about the same time each day. Others can be more flexible with the timing of their meals. Depending on your diabetes medicines or type of insulin, you may need to eat the same amount of carbohydrates at the same time each day. If you take "mealtime" insulin, your eating schedule can be more flexible.

If you use certain diabetes medicines or insulin and you skip or delay a meal, your blood glucose level can drop too low. Ask your health care team when you should eat and whether you should eat before and after physical activity.

How much can I eat if I have diabetes?

Eating the right amount of food will also help you manage your blood glucose level and your weight. Your health care team can help you figure out how much food and how many calories you should eat each day. Look up how many calories are in what you eat and drink at the USDA's Food-A-Pedia.

Weight-loss planning

If you are overweight or obese, work with your health care team to create a weight-loss plan.

These tools may help: The Body Weight Planner can help you tailor your plans to reach and maintain your goal weight.

The SuperTracker lets you track your food, physical activity, and weight.

To lose weight, you need to eat fewer calories and replace less healthy foods with foods lower in calories, fat, and sugar.

If you have diabetes, are overweight or obese, and are planning to have a baby, you should try to lose any excess weight before you become pregnant.

Why should I be physically active if I have diabetes?

Physical activity is an important part of managing your blood glucose level and staying healthy. Being active has many health benefits.

Physical activity

- lowers blood glucose levels

- lowers blood pressure

- improves blood flow

- burns extra calories so you can keep your weight down if needed

- improves your mood

- can prevent falls and improve memory in the elderly

How can I be physically active safely if I have diabetes?

Be sure to drink water before, during, and after exercise to stay well hydrated. The following are some other tips for safe physical activity when you have diabetes.

Drink water when you exercise to stay well hydrated.

Plan ahead

Talk with your health care team before you start a new exercise routine, especially if you have other health problems. Your health care team will tell you a target range for your blood glucose level and suggest how you can be active safely.

Your health care team also can help you decide the best time of day for you to do physical activity based on your daily schedule, meal plan, and diabetes medicines. If you take insulin, you need to balance the activity that you do with your insulin doses and meals so you don't get low blood glucose.

Prevent low blood glucose

Because physical activity lowers your blood glucose, you should protect yourself against low blood glucose levels, also called hypoglycemia. You are most likely to have hypoglycemia if you take insulin or certain other diabetes medicines, such as a sulfonylurea. Hypoglycemia also can occur after a long intense workout or if you have skipped a meal before being active. Hypoglycemia can happen during or up to 24 hours after physical activity.

Planning is key to preventing hypoglycemia. For instance, if you take insulin, your health care provider might suggest you take less insulin or eat a small snack with carbohydrates before, during, or after physical activity, especially intense activity.

You may need to check your blood glucose level before, during, and right after you are physically active.

Stay safe when blood glucose is highIf you have type 1 diabetes, avoid vigorous physical activity when you have ketones in your blood or urine. Ketones are chemicals your body might make when your blood glucose level is too high, a condition called hyperglycemia, and your insulin level is too low. If you are physically active when you have ketones in your blood or urine, your blood glucose level may go even higher. Ask your health care team what level of ketones are dangerous for you and how to test for them. Ketones are uncommon in people with type 2 diabetes.

Take care of your feet

People with diabetes may have problems with their feet because of poor blood flow and nerve damage that can result from high blood glucose levels. To help prevent foot problems, you should wear comfortable, supportive shoes and take care of your feet before, during, and after physical activity.

What physical activities should I do if I have diabetes?

Most kinds of physical activity can help you take care of your diabetes. Certain activities may be unsafe for some people, such as those with low vision or nerve damage to their feet. Ask your health care team what physical activities are safe for you. Many people choose walking with friends or family members for their activity.

Doing different types of physical activity each week will give you the most health benefits. Mixing it up also helps reduce boredom and lower your chance of getting hurt. Try these options for physical activity.

Add extra activity to your daily routine If you have been inactive or you are trying a new activity, start slowly, with 5 to 10 minutes a day. Then add a little more time each week. Increase daily activity by spending less time in front of a TV or other screens. Try these simple ways to add physical activities in your life each day:

Walk around while you talk on the phone or during TV commercials.

Do chores, such as work in the garden, rake leaves, clean the house, or wash the car.

Park at the far end of the shopping center, parking lot and walk to the store.

Take the stairs instead of the elevator.

Make your family outings active, such as a family bike ride or a walk in a park.

If you are sitting for a long time, such as working at a desk or watching TV, do some light activity for 3 minutes or more every half hour.6 Light activities include

- leg lifts or extensions

- overhead arm stretches

- desk chair swivels

- torso twists

- side lunges

- walking in place

Do aerobic exercise

Aerobic exercise is activity that makes your heart beat faster and makes you breathe harder. You should aim for doing aerobic exercise for 30 minutes a day most days of the week. You do not have to do all the activity at one time. You can split up these minutes into a few times throughout the day.

To get the most out of your activity, exercise at a moderate to vigorous level. Try

- walking briskly or hiking

- climbing stairs

- swimming or a water-aerobics class

- dancing

- riding a bicycle or a stationary bicycle

- taking an exercise class

- playing basketball, tennis, or other sports

Talk with your health care team about how to warm up and cool down before and after you exercise.

Do strength training to build muscle

Strength training is a light or moderate physical activity that builds muscle and helps keep your bones healthy. Strength training is important for both men and women. When you have more muscle and less body fat, you'll burn more calories. Burning more calories can help you lose and keep off extra weight.

You can do strength training with hand weights, elastic bands, or weight machines. Try to do strength training two to three times a week. Start with a light weight. Slowly increase the size of your weights as your muscles become stronger.

You can do strength training with hand weights, elastic bands, or weight machines.

Do stretching exercises

Stretching exercises are light or moderate physical activity. When you stretch, you increase your flexibility, lower your stress, and help prevent sore muscles.

You can choose from many types of stretching exercises. Yoga is a type of stretching that focuses on your breathing and helps you relax. Even if you have problems moving or balancing, certain types of yoga can help. For instance, chair yoga has stretches you can do when sitting in a chair or holding onto a chair while standing. Your health care team can suggest whether yoga is right for you.

TREATMENT FOR TYPE 2 DIABETES

You can effectively manage type 2 diabetes. Your doctor will tell you how often you should check your blood glucose levels. The goal is to stay within a specific range.

Follow these tips to manage type 2 diabetes:

Include foods rich in fiber and healthy carbohydrates in your diet. Eating fruits, vegetables, and whole grains will help keep your blood glucose levels steady.

- Eat at regular intervals

- Only eat until you're full.

- Control your weight and keep your heart healthy.

That means keeping refined carbohydrates, sweets, and animal fats to a minimum.

- Get about half an hour of aerobic activity daily to help keep your heart healthy.

- Exercise helps to control blood glucose, too.

Your doctor will explain how to recognize the early symptoms of blood sugar that's too high or too low and what to do in each situation. Your doctor will also help you learn which foods are healthy and which foods aren't.

Not everyone with type 2 diabetes needs to use insulin. If you do, it's because your pancreas isn't making enough insulin on its own. It's crucial that you take insulin as directed. There are other prescription medications that may help as well.

In addition, many people with type 2 diabetes require oral medication, insulin, or both to control their blood glucose levels. People with diabetes must take responsibility for their day-to-day care, and keep blood glucose levels from going too low or too high.

People with diabetes should see a health care provider who will monitor their diabetes control and help them learn to manage their diabetes. In addition, people with diabetes may see endocrinologists, who may specialize in diabetes care; ophthalmologists for eye examinations; podiatrists for routine foot care; and dietitians and diabetes educators who teach the skills needed for daily diabetes management.

CAUSES OF TYPE 2 DIABETES

Insulin is a naturally occurring hormone. Your pancreas produces it and releases it when you eat. Insulin helps transport sugar from your bloodstream to cells throughout your body, where it's used for energy.

If you have type 2 diabetes, your body becomes resistant to insulin. Your body is no longer using the hormone efficiently. This forces your pancreas to work harder to make more insulin. Over time, this can damage cells in your pancreas. Eventually, your pancreas may not be able to produce any insulin.

If you don't produce enough insulin or if your body doesn't use it efficiently, glucose builds up in your bloodstream. This leaves your body's cells starved for energy.

Doctors don't know exactly what triggers this series of events.

It may have to do with cell dysfunction in the pancreas or with cell signaling and regulation. In some people, the liver produces too much glucose. There may be a genetic predisposition to developing type 2 diabetes.

There's also a genetic predisposition to obesity, which increases the risk of insulin resistance and diabetes. There could also be an environmental trigger.

Most likely, it's a combination of factors that increases the risk of type 2 diabetes. Research into the causes of type 2 diabetes is ongoing.

Type 2 diabetes—the most common form of diabetes—is caused by several factors, including lifestyle factors and genes.

Overweight, obesity, and physical inactivity. You are more likely to develop type 2 diabetes if you are not physically active and are overweight or obese. Extra weight sometimes causes insulin resistance and is common in people with type 2 diabetes. The location of body fat also makes a difference. Extra belly fat is linked to insulin resistance, type 2 diabetes, and heart and blood vessel disease. To see if your weight puts you at risk for type 2 diabetes, check out these Body Mass Index (BMI) charts.

INSULIN RESISTANCE

Type 2 diabetes usually begins with insulin resistance, a condition in which muscle, liver, and fat cells do not use insulin well. As a result, your body needs more insulin to help glucose enter cells. At first, the pancreas makes more insulin to keep up with the added demand. Over time, the pancreas can't make enough insulin, and blood glucose levels rise.

Genes and family history

As in type 1 diabetes, certain genes may make you more likely to develop type 2 diabetes. The disease tends to run in families and occurs more often in these racial/ethnic groups:

African Americans

Alaska Natives

American Indians

Asian Americans

Hispanics/Latinos

Native Hawaiians

Pacific Islanders

Genes also can increase the risk of type 2 diabetes by increasing a person's tendency to become overweight or obese.

MEDICATIONS FOR TYPE 2 DIABETES

In some cases, lifestyle changes are enough to keep type 2 diabetes under control. If not, there are several medications that may help. Some of these medications are:

Metformin, which can lower your blood sugar levels and improve how your body responds to insulin. Sulfonylureas, which help your body make more insulin. Meglitinides or glinides, which are fast-acting, short-duration medications that stimulate your pancreas to release more insulin. Thiazolidinediones, which make your body more sensitive to insulin. Dipeptidyl peptidase-4 inhibitors, which are milder medications that help reduce blood sugar levels. Glucagon-like peptide-1 receptor agonists, which slow digestion and improve blood sugar levels. Sodium-glucose cotransporter-2 inhibitors, which help prevent the kidneys from reabsorbing sugar into the blood and sending it out in your urine

Each of these medications can cause side effects. It may take some time to find the best medication or combination of medications to treat your diabetes.

If your blood pressure or cholesterol levels are a problem, you may need medications to address those needs as well.

If your body can't make enough insulin, you may need insulin therapy. You may only need a long-acting injection you can take at night or you may need to take insulin several times per day.

Insulin, Medicines, & Other Diabetes Treatments

Taking insulin or other diabetes medicines is often part of treating diabetes. Along with healthy food choices and physical activity, medicine can help you manage the disease. Some other treatment options are also available.

What medicines might I take for diabetes?

The medicine you take will vary by your type of diabetes and how well the medicine controls your blood glucose levels, also called blood sugar. Other factors, such as your other health conditions, medication costs, and your daily schedule may play a role in what diabetes medicine you take.

Type 2 diabetes

Some people with type 2 diabetes can manage their disease by making healthy food choices and being more physically active. Many people with type 2 diabetes need diabetes medicines as well. These medicines may include diabetes pills or medicines you inject under your skin, such as insulin. In time, you may need more than one diabetes medicine to control your blood glucose. Even if you do not take insulin, you may need it at special times, such as during pregnancy or if you are in the hospital.

What are the different types of insulin?

Several types of insulin are available. Each type starts to work at a different speed, known as "onset," and its effects last a different length of time, known as "duration." Most types of insulin reach a peak, which is when they have the strongest effect. Then the effects of the insulin wear off over the next few hours or so.

What are the different ways to take insulin?

The way you take insulin may depend on your lifestyle, insurance plan, and preferences. You may decide that needles are not for you and prefer a different method. Talk with your doctor about the options and which is best for you. Most people with diabetes use a needle and syringe, pen, or insulin pump. Inhalers, injection ports, and jet injectors are less common.

Needle and syringe

You'll give yourself insulin shots using a needle and syringe. You will draw up your dose of insulin from the vial, or bottle, into the syringe. Insulin works fastest when you inject it in your belly, but you should rotate spots where you inject insulin. Other injection spots include your thigh, buttocks, or upper arm. Some people with diabetes who take insulin need two to four shots a day to reach their blood glucose targets. Others can take a single shot.

An insulin pen looks like a pen but has a needle for its point. Some insulin pens come filled with insulin and are disposable. Others have room for an insulin cartridge that you insert and then replace after use. Insulin pens cost more than needles and syringes but many people find them easier to use.

An insulin pump is a small machine that gives you small, steady doses of insulin throughout the day. You wear one type of pump outside your body on a belt or in a pocket or pouch. The insulin pump connects to a small plastic tube and a very small needle. You insert the needle under your skin and it stays in place for several days. Insulin then pumps from the machine through the tube into your body 24 hours a day. You also can give yourself doses of insulin through the pump at mealtimes. Another type of pump has no tubes and attaches directly to your skin, such as a self-adhesive pod.

Inhaler

Another way to take insulin is by breathing powdered insulin from an inhaler device into your mouth. The insulin goes into your lungs and moves quickly into your blood. Inhaled insulin is only for adults with type 1 or type 2 diabetes.

Injection port

An injection port has a short tube that you insert into the tissue beneath your skin. On the skin's surface, an adhesive patch or dressing holds the port in place. You inject insulin through the port with a needle and syringe or an insulin pen. The port stays in place for a few days, and then you replace the port. With an injection port, you no longer puncture your skin for each shot— only when you apply a new port.

Jet injector

This device sends a fine spray of insulin into the skin at high pressure instead of using a needle to deliver the insulin.

What oral medicines treat type 2 diabetes?

You may need medicines along with healthy eating and physical activity habits to manage your type 2 diabetes. You can take many diabetes medicines by mouth. These medicines are called oral medicines.

Most people with type 2 diabetes start medical treatment with metformin pills. Metformin also comes as a liquid. Metformin lowers the amount of glucose that your liver makes and helps your body use insulin better. This drug may help you lose a small amount of weight.

Other oral medicines act in different ways to lower blood glucose levels. You may need to add another diabetes medicine after a while or use a combination treatment. Combining two or three kinds of diabetes medicines can lower blood glucose levels more than taking just one.

What other injectable medicines treat type 2 diabetes?

Besides insulin, other types of injected medicines are available. These medicines help keep your blood glucose level from going too high after you eat. They may make you feel less hungry and help you lose some weight. Other injectable medicines are not substitutes for insulin. Learn more about noninsulin injectable medicines.

What should I know about side effects of diabetes medicines?

Side effects are problems that result from a medicine. Some diabetes medicines can cause hypoglycemia, also called low blood glucose, if you don't balance your medicines with food and activity.

Ask your doctor whether your diabetes medicine can cause hypoglycemia or other side effects, such as upset stomach and weight gain. Take your diabetes medicines as your health care professional has instructed you, to help prevent side effects and diabetes problems.

Do I have other treatment options for my diabetes?

When medicines and lifestyle changes are not enough to manage your diabetes, a less common treatment may be an option. Other treatments include bariatric surgery for certain people with type 1 or type 2 diabetes, and an "artificial pancreas" and pancreatic islet transplantation for some people with type 1 diabetes.

Bariatric surgery

Also called weight-loss surgery or metabolic surgery, bariatric surgery may help some people with obesity and type 2 diabetes lose a large amount of weight and regain normal blood glucose levels. Some people with diabetes may no longer need their diabetes medicine after bariatric surgery. Whether and for how long blood glucose levels improve seems to vary by the patient, type of weight-loss surgery, and the amount of weight the person loses. Other factors include how long someone has had diabetes and whether or not the person uses insulin.

Recent research suggests that weight-loss surgery also may help improve blood glucose control in people with type 1 diabetes who are obese. Researchers are studying the long-term results of bariatric surgery in people with type 1 and type 2 diabetes.

Artificial Pancreas

The NIDDK has played an important role in developing "artificial pancreas" technology. An artificial pancreas replaces manual blood glucose testing and the use of insulin shots or a pump. A single system monitors blood glucose levels around the clock and provides insulin or a combination of insulin and a second hormone, glucagon, automatically. The system can also be monitored remotely, for example by parents or medical staff.

TYPE 2 DIABETES IN CHILDREN

Type 2 diabetes in children is a growing problem. According to the American Diabetes Association, approximately 208,000 Americans under age 20 have diabetes.

The reasons for this are complex, but risk factors include: being overweight, or having a body mass index above the 85th percentile having a birth weight of 9 pounds or more being born to a mother who had diabetes while she was pregnant having a close family member with type 2 diabetes having a sedentary lifestyle being American Indian, Alaska Native, African-American, Asian-American, Latino, or Pacific Islander

The symptoms of type 2 diabetes in children include:

- excessive thirst

- excessive hunger

- increased urination

- sores that are slow to heal

- frequent infections

- Fatigue

- blurry vision

- areas of darkened skin

See your child's doctor immediately if your child has symptoms of diabetes. Untreated diabetes can lead to serious and even life-threatening complications.

A random blood sugar test may reveal high blood sugar levels. A hemoglobin A1C test can provide more information about average blood sugar levels over a few months. Your child may also need a fasting blood sugar test.

If your child's doctor diagnoses them with diabetes, your doctor will need to determine if it's type 1 or type 2 before suggesting a specific treatment.

You can help lower your child's risk by encouraging them to eat well and to be physically active every day.

RISK FACTORS FOR TYPE 2 DIABETES

We may not understand the exact causes of type 2 diabetes, but we do know that certain factors can put you at increased risk.

Certain factors are out of your control:

- Your risk is greater if you have a brother, sister, or parent who has type 2 diabetes.

- You can develop type 2 diabetes at any age, but your risk increases as you get older.

- Your risk is particularly high after age 45.

You may be able to change these factors:

Being overweight means that you have more fatty tissue, which makes your cells more resistant to insulin. Extra fat in the abdomen increases your risk more than extra fat in the hips and thighs.

- Your risk increases if you have a sedentary lifestyle.

- Regular exercise uses up glucose and helps your cells respond better to insulin.

- Eating a lot of junk foods or eating too much wreaks havoc on your blood glucose levels.

- You're also at increased risk if you've had gestational diabetes or if you have prediabetes.

Additional Risk Factors for Type 2 Diabetes

Your chances of developing type 2 diabetes depend on a combination of risk factors such as your genes and lifestyle. Although you can't change risk factors such as family history, age, or ethnicity, you can change lifestyle risk factors around eating, physical activity, and weight. These lifestyle changes can affect your chances of developing type 2 diabetes.

Read about risk factors for type 2 diabetes below and see which ones apply to you. Taking action on the factors you can change can help you delay or prevent type 2 diabetes.

You are more likely to develop type 2 diabetes if you are overweight or obese are age 45 or older have a family history of diabetes are African American, Alaska Native, American Indian, Asian American, Hispanic/Latino, Native Hawaiian, or Pacific Islander have high blood pressure have a low level of HDL ("good") cholesterol, or a high level of triglycerides have a history of gestational diabetes or gave birth to a baby weighing 9 pounds or more are not physically active, have a history of heart disease or stroke, have depression or have polycystic ovary syndrome, also called.

PCOS: have acanthosis nigricans—dark, thick, and velvety skin around your neck or armpits. You can also take the Diabetes Risk Test to learn about your risk for type 2 diabetes.

To see if your weight puts you at risk for type 2 diabetes, find your height in the Body Mass Index (BMI) charts below. If your weight is equal to or more than the weight listed, you have a greater chance of developing the disease.

If you are not Asian American or Pacific Islander   If you are Asian American   If you are Pacific Islander

At-risk BMI ≥ 25		At-risk BMI ≥ 23		At-risk BMI ≥ 26	
Height	Weight	Height	Weight	Height	Weight
4'10"	119	4'10"	110	4'10"	124
4'11"	124	4'11"	114	4'11"	128
5'0"	128	5'0"	118	5'0"	133
5'1"	132	5'1"	122	5'1"	137
5'2"	136	5'2"	126	5'2"	142
5'3"	141	5'3"	130	5'3"	146
5'4"	145	5'4"	134	5'4"	151
5'5"	150	5'5"	138	5'5"	156
5'6"	155	5'6"	142	5'6"	161
5'7"	159	5'7"	146	5'7"	166
5'8"	164	5'8"	151	5'8"	171
5'9"	169	5'9"	155	5'9"	176
5'10"	174	5'10"	160	5'10"	181
5'11"	179	5'11"	165	5'11"	186
6'0"	184	6'0"	169	6'0"	191
6'1"	189	6'1"	174	6'1"	197
6'2"	194	6'2"	179	6'2"	202
6'3"	200	6'3"	184	6'3"	208
6'4"	205	6'4"	189	6'4"	213

TIPS FOR HOW TO PREVENT TYPE 2 DIABETES

You can't always prevent type 2 diabetes. There's nothing you can do about your genetics, ethnicity, or age.

If you have prediabetes or other diabetes risk factors and even if you don't, a few lifestyle tweaks can help delay or even prevent the onset of type 2 diabetes. These changes in diet, exercise, and weight management work together to help keep your blood sugar levels within the ideal range all day long:

• Diet

Your diet should be high in nutrient-rich carbohydrates and fiber. You also need heart-healthy omega-3 fatty acids from certain kinds of fish and monounsaturated and polyunsaturated fats. Dairy products should be low in fat. It's not only what you eat, but also how much you eat that matters. You should be careful about portion sizes and try to eat meals at about the same time every day.

• Exercise

Type 2 diabetes is associated with inactivity. Getting 30 minutes of aerobic exercise every day can improve your overall health. Try to add in extra movement throughout the day, too.

• Weight management

You're more likely to develop type 2 diabetes if you're overweight. Eating a healthy, balanced diet and getting daily exercise should help you keep your weight under control. If those changes aren't working, your doctor can make some recommendations for losing weight safely.

You can take steps to help prevent or delay type 2 diabetes by losing weight if you are overweight, eating fewer calories, and being more physically active. Talk with your health care professional about any of the health conditions listed above that may require medical treatment. Managing these health problems may help reduce your chances of developing type 2 diabetes. Also, ask your health care professional about any medicines you take that might increase your risk.

Perhaps you have learned that you have a high chance of developing type 2 diabetes, the most common type of diabetes. You might be overweight or have a parent, brother, or sister with type 2 diabetes. Maybe you had gestational diabetes, which is diabetes that develops during pregnancy. These are just a few examples of factors that can raise your chances of developing type 2 diabetes.

Diabetes can cause serious health problems, such as heart disease, stroke, and eye and foot problems. Prediabetes also can cause health problems. The good news is that type 2 diabetes can be delayed or even prevented. The longer you have diabetes, the more likely you are to develop health problems, so delaying diabetes by even a few years will benefit your health. You can help prevent or delay type 2 diabetes by losing a modest amount of weight by following a reduced-calorie eating plan and being physically active most days of the week. Ask your doctor if you should take the diabetes drug metformin to help prevent or delay type 2 diabetes.

Research such as the Diabetes Prevention Program shows that you can do a lot to reduce your chances of developing type 2 diabetes.

Here are some things you can change to lower your risk:

- Lose weight and keep it off.

- You may be able to prevent or delay diabetes by losing 5 to 7 percent of your starting weight.1 For instance, if you weigh 200 pounds, your goal would be to lose about 10 to 14 pounds.

- Move more. Get at least 30 minutes of physical activity 5 days a week. If you have not been active, talk with your health care professional about which activities are best.

- Start slowly to build up to your goal.

- Eat healthy foods most of the time.

- Eat smaller portions to reduce the amount of calories you eat each day and help you lose weight.

- Choosing foods with less fat is another way to reduce calories.

- Drink water instead of sweetened beverages.

- Ask your health care professional about what other changes you can make to prevent or delay type 2 diabetes.

Most often, your best chance for preventing type 2 diabetes is to make lifestyle changes that work for you long term. Get started with Your Game Plan to Prevent Type 2 Diabetes.

Prediabetes is when your blood glucose, also called blood sugar, levels are higher than normal, but not high enough to be called diabetes. Having prediabetes is serious because it raises your chance of developing type 2 diabetes. Many of the same factors that raise your chance of developing type 2 diabetes put you at risk for prediabetes.

Other names for prediabetes include impaired fasting glucose or impaired glucose tolerance. Some people call prediabetes "borderline diabetes."

About 1 in 3 Americans has prediabetes, according to recent diabetes statistics from the Centers for Disease Control and Prevention. You won't know if you have prediabetes unless you are tested. If you have prediabetes, you can lower your chance of developing type 2 diabetes. Lose weight if you need to, become more physically active, and follow a reduced-calorie eating plan.

Get started with Your Game Plan to Prevent Type 2 Diabetes. For more support, you can find a lifestyle change program near you through the National Diabetes Prevention Program.

Photo of two smiling middle-aged women on exercise bikes Being physically active is one way to help prevent prediabetes from progressing to type 2 diabetes.

PREVENTING DIABETES PROBLEMS

Heart Disease & Stroke

Diabetes can damage blood vessels and lead to heart disease and stroke. You can do a lot to prevent heart disease and stroke by managing your blood glucose, blood pressure, and cholesterol levels; and by not smoking.

Low Blood Glucose (Hypoglycemia) Hypoglycemia occurs when your blood glucose drops too low. Certain diabetes medicines make low blood glucose more likely. You can prevent hypoglycemia by following your meal plan and balancing your physical activity, food, and medicines. Testing your blood glucose regularly can also help prevent hypoglycemia.

Nerve Damage (Diabetic Neuropathy) Diabetic neuropathy is nerve damage that can result from diabetes. Different types of nerve damage affect different parts of your body. Managing your diabetes can help prevent nerve damage that affects your feet and limbs, and organs such as your heart.

Kidney Disease

Diabetic kidney disease also called diabetic nephropathy, is a kidney disease caused by diabetes. You can help protect your kidneys by managing your diabetes and meeting your blood pressure goals.

Foot Problems

Diabetes can cause nerve damage and poor blood flow, which can lead to serious foot problems. Common foot problems, such as a callus, can lead to pain or an infection that makes it hard to walk. Get a foot checkup at each visit with your health care team.

Eye Disease

Diabetes can damage your eyes and lead to eye problems such as low vision and blindness. The best way to prevent diabetes-related eye disease is to manage your blood glucose, blood pressure, and cholesterol; and to not smoke. Also, have a dilated eye exam once a year. Finding eye disease early can help prevent vision loss.

Gum Disease & Other Dental Problems

Diabetes can lead to problems in your mouth, such as infection, gum disease, or dry mouth. To help keep your mouth healthy, manage your blood glucose, brush your teeth twice a day, see your dentist at least once a year, and don't smoke.

Sexual & Urologic Problems

Having diabetes can increase your chance of having bladder problems and changes in sexual function.

Following your diabetes management plan is important to help prevent or delay sexual and urologic problems.

Depression & Diabetes

Depression is common among people with a chronic, or long-term, illness such as diabetes. Depression can be treated so tell your doctor if you feel sad, hopeless, or anxious.

Cancer & Diabetes

Diabetes is linked to some types of cancer. Many risk factors for cancer and for diabetes are the same. Not smoking and getting recommended cancer screenings can help prevent cancer.

Dementia & Diabetes

High blood glucose increases the chance of developing dementia. Tell your doctor if you are forgetful because dementia can make it hard to manage your diabetes.

Sleep Apnea & Diabetes

People who have sleep apnea —when you stop breathing for short periods during sleep—are more likely to develop type 2 diabetes. Sleep apnea also can make diabetes worse. Treatment for sleep apnea can help.

RECEIVING A TYPE 2 DIABETES DIAGNOSIS

Whether or not you have prediabetes, you should see your doctor right away if you have the symptoms of diabetes. Your doctor can get a lot of information from blood work. Diagnostic testing may include the following:

A hemoglobin A1C test is also called a glycosylated hemoglobin test. It measures average blood glucose levels for the previous two or three months. You don't need to fast for this test, and your doctor can diagnose you based on the results.

You need to fast for eight hours before having a fasting plasma glucose test. This test measures how much glucose is in your plasma.

During an oral glucose tolerance test, your blood is drawn before and two hours after you drink a dose of glucose. The test results show how well your body deals with glucose before and after the drink.

If you have diabetes, your doctor will provide you with information about how to manage the disease, including:

- how to monitor blood glucose levels on your own

- dietary recommendations

- physical activity recommendations

- information about any medications that you need

You may need to see an endocrinologist who specializes in the treatment of diabetes. You'll probably need to visit your doctor more often at first to make sure your treatment plan is working.

Diabetes Tests & Diagnosis

Your health care professional can diagnose diabetes, prediabetes, and gestational diabetes through blood tests. The blood tests show if your blood glucose, also called blood sugar, is too high.

Do not try to diagnose yourself if you think you might have diabetes. Testing equipment that you can buy over the counter, such as a blood glucose meter, cannot diagnose diabetes.

Who should be tested for diabetes?

Anyone who has symptoms of diabetes should be tested for the disease. Some people will not have any symptoms, but may have risk factors for diabetes and need to be tested. Testing allows health care professionals to find diabetes sooner and work with their patients to manage diabetes and prevent complications.

Testing also allows health care professionals to find prediabetes. Making lifestyle changes to lose a modest amount of weight if you are overweight may help you delay or prevent type 2 diabetes.

Type 1 diabetes

Most often, testing for type 1 diabetes occurs in people with diabetes symptoms. Doctors usually diagnose type 1 diabetes in children and young adults. Because type 1 diabetes can run in families, a study called TrialNet offers free testing to family members of people with the disease, even if they don't have symptoms.

Type 2 diabetes

Experts recommend routine testing for type 2 diabetes if you are age 45 or older are between the ages of 19 and 44, are overweight or obese, and have one or more other diabetes risk factor are a woman who had gestational diabetes1

Medicare covers the cost of diabetes tests for people with certain risk factors for diabetes. If you have Medicare, find out if you qualify for coverage. If you have different insurance, ask your insurance company if it covers diabetes tests.

Though type 2 diabetes most often develops in adults, children also can develop type 2 diabetes. Experts recommend testing children between the ages of 10 and 18 who are overweight or obese and have at least two other risk factors for developing diabetes. low birthweight a mother who had diabetes while pregnant with them any risk factor mentioned in Risk Factors for Type 2 Diabetes

Gestational diabetes

All pregnant women who do not have a prior diabetes diagnosis should be tested for gestational diabetes. If you are pregnant, you will take a glucose challenge test between 24 and 28 weeks of pregnancy.

How is Diabetes Diagnosed?

There are several types of tests that can be used to diagnose diabetes or pre-diabetes:

- Fasting Plasma Glucose Test (FPG),

- Oral Glucose Tolerance Test (OGTT)

- a random non-fasting plasma glucose test

- and a hemoglobin A1c test.

Any test should be repeated on at least two occasions. With two or more tests you can be sure the result is accurate. a doctor is a person who can diagnose diabetes

According to the American Diabetes Association, a FPG test that results in a fasting blood glucose level between 100 and 125 mg/dl signals pre-diabetes (or 5.6 mmol/l and 6.9 mmol/l). A person with a fasting blood glucose level of 126 mg/dl or higher has diabetes (or 7.0 mmol/l).

In the OGTT, a person's blood glucose level is measured after a fast and two hours after drinking a glucose-rich beverage. If the two-hour blood glucose level is between 140 and 199 mg/dl (7.8 mmol/l and 11.1 mmol/l), the person tested has pre-diabetes. If the two-hour blood glucose level is 200 mg/dl or higher, the person tested has diabetes.

A random, non-fasting blood glucose of 200 mg/dL or higher may indicate diabetes (11.1 mmol/l). Symptoms of increased urination, increase thirst, and unexplained weight loss would support a diagonsis of diabetes. The random test is usually followed by either FPG or OGT for confirmation.

The hemoglobin A1c test measures the level of glucose in your blood for the past three months. Two hemoglobin A1c values greater than 6.5% would diagnose diabetes. If one value is above 6.5% and one is below 6.5%, an FBG or OGT is usually ordered by the doctor. Having values between 5.7% and 6.4% is pre-diabetes.

What is Pre-diabetes?

Pre-diabetes occurs when blood glucose levels are higher than normal, but lower than levels used to diagnose diabetes. Other phrases sometimes used to describe pre-diabetes include "borderline diabetes" or "blood sugar a little high." People with pre-diabetes are said to have impaired glucose tolerance and/or impaired fasting glucose levels.

The American Diabetes Association defines impaired glucose tolerance and impaired fasting glucose as:

• Impaired Glucose Tolerance

Impaired Glucose Tolerance is a 2-hour value of an oral glucose tolerance test that is greater than orequal to 140 mg/dl but less than 200 mg/dl. Impaired Glucose Tolerance Diagnostic categories of oral glucose tolerance tests.

• Impaired Fasting Glucose

Impaired Fasting Glucose is a fasting blood glucose level of greater than or equal to 100mg/dl but less than 126 mg/dl. Impaired Fasting Glucose Diagnostic categories of impaired fasting blood glucose tests.

Pre-diabetes puts people at high risk for developing diabetes, but also gives them a head start on preventing this disease. People told that they have pre-diabetes can often bring their blood glucose levels back down to normal by balancing a healthy diet with physical activity and weight loss.

Can People with Diabetes Prevent the Complications of this Disease?

Diabetes is a serious disease that can affect the heart, circulation, eyes, feet, kidneys, nervous system, teeth, and gums. Diabetes affects so many organs and systems, because blood travels throughout the whole body. When blood glucose becomes too high, it can damage the blood vessels of the body and lead to cardiovascular disease (heart), retinopathy (eyes), amputations (legs and feet), kidney disease, neuropathy (nervous system), and impotence (sexual function).

With the exception of the heart, high blood glucose damages these other organs because small blood vessels keep the organs working. The high blood glucose can damage these tiny blood vessels. When these are damaged, the oxygen, nutrients, and cell communication doesn't work normally. This leads to retinopathy (eyes), amputations (legs and feet), kidney disease, neuropathy (nervous system), and impotence (sexual function). The high blood glucose in the heart can increase fatty deposits and lead to cardiovascular disease. risk of complications can be greatly reduced by keeping blood glucose levels within the target range

The risk of these complications can be greatly reduced by keeping blood glucose levels within the target range. For this reason, it is important to check blood glucose levels every day, and share these values with a health care provider.

Health care professionals most often use the fasting plasma glucose (FPG) test or the A1C test to diagnose diabetes. In some cases, they may use a random plasma glucose (RPG) test.

Fasting plasma glucose (FPG) test The FPG blood test measures your blood glucose level at a single point in time. For the most reliable results, it is best to have this test in the morning, after you fast for at least 8 hours. Fasting means having nothing to eat or drink except sips of water.

A1C test

The A1C test is a blood test that provides your average levels of blood glucose over the past 3 months. Other names for the A1C test are hemoglobin A1C, HbA1C, glycated hemoglobin, and glycosylated hemoglobin test. You can eat and drink before this test. When it comes to using the A1C to diagnose diabetes, your doctor will consider factors such as your age and whether you have anemia or another problem with your blood. The A1C test is not accurate in people with anemia. Your health care professional will report your A1C test result as a percentage, such as an A1C of 7 percent. The higher the percentage, the higher your average blood glucose levels. People with diabetes also use information from the A1C test to help manage their diabetes.

Random plasma glucose (RPG) test.

Sometimes health care professionals use the RPG test to diagnose diabetes when diabetes symptoms are present and they do not want to wait until you have fasted. You do not need to fast overnight for the RPG test. You may have this blood test at any time.

What tests are used to diagnose gestational diabetes?

Pregnant women may have the glucose challenge test, the oral glucose tolerance test, or both. These tests show how well your body handles glucose.

Glucose challenge test

If you are pregnant and a health care professional is checking you for gestational diabetes, you may first receive the glucose challenge test. Another name for this test is the glucose screening test. In this test, a health care professional will draw your blood 1 hour after you drink a sweet liquid containing glucose. You do not need to fast for this test. If your blood glucose is too high—135 to 140 or more—you may need to return for an oral glucose tolerance test while fasting.

Oral glucose tolerance test (OGTT)

The OGTT measures blood glucose after you fast for at least 8 hours. First, a health care professional will draw your blood. Then you will drink the liquid containing glucose. For diagnosing gestational diabetes, you will need your blood drawn every hour for 2 to 3 hours.

High blood glucose levels at any two or more blood test times during the OGTT—fasting, 1 hour, 2 hours, or 3 hours—mean you have gestational diabetes. Your health care team will explain what your OGTT results mean.

Health care professionals also can use the OGTT to diagnose type 2 diabetes and prediabetes in people who are not pregnant. The OGTT helps health care professionals detect type 2 diabetes and prediabetes better than the FPG test. However, the OGTT is a more expensive test and is not as easy to give. To diagnose type 2 diabetes and prediabetes, a health care professional will need to draw your blood 1 hour after you drink the liquid containing glucose and again after 2 hours.

What test numbers tell me if I have diabetes or prediabetes?

Each test to detect diabetes and prediabetes uses a different measurement. Usually, the same test method needs to be repeated on a second day to diagnose diabetes. Your doctor may also use a second test method to confirm that you have diabetes.

what kind of diabetes I have?

Even though the tests described here can confirm that you have diabetes, they can't identify what type you have. Sometimes health care professionals are unsure if diabetes is type 1 or type 2. A rare type of diabetes that can occur in babies, called monogenic diabetes, can also be mistaken for type 1 diabetes. Treatment depends on the type of diabetes, so knowing which type you have is important.

To find out if your diabetes is type 1, your health care professional may look for certain autoantibodies. Autoantibodies are antibodies that mistakenly attack your healthy tissues and cells. The presence of one or more of several types of autoantibodies specific to diabetes is common in type 1 diabetes, but not in type 2 or monogenic diabetes. A health care professional will have to draw your blood for this test.

If you had diabetes while you were pregnant, you should get tested 6 to 12 weeks after your baby is born to see if you have type 2 diabetes.

COMPLICATIONS ASSOCIATED WITH TYPE 2 DIABETES

For many people, type 2 diabetes can be effectively managed. It can affect virtually all your organs and lead to serious complications, including:

- skin problems, such as bacterial or fungal Infections

- nerve damage, or neuropathy, which can cause a loss of sensation or numbness and tingling in your extremities as well as digestive issues, such as vomiting, diarrhea, and constipation poor circulation to the feet, which makes it hard for your feet to heal when you have a cut or an infection and can also lead to gangrene and loss of the foot or leg

- hearing impairment

- retinal damage, or retinopathy, and eye damage, which can cause deteriorating vision, glaucoma, and cataracts

- cardiovascular diseases such as high blood pressure, narrowing of the arteries, angina, heart attack, and stroke, kidney damage and kidney failure

Hypoglycemia

Hypoglycemia can occur when your blood sugar is low. The symptoms can include shakiness, dizziness, and difficulty speaking. You can usually remedy this by having a "quick-fix" food or drink, such as fruit juice, a soft drink, or a hard candy.

Hyperglycemia

Hyperglycemia can happen when blood sugar is high. It's typically characterized by frequent urination and increased thirst. Exercising can help lower your blood sugar level.

Complications during and after pregnancy

If you have diabetes while you're pregnant, you'll need to monitor your condition carefully. Diabetes that's poorly controlled can:

- complicate labor and delivery

- harm your baby's developing organs

- cause your baby to gain too much weight

- increase your baby's risk of developing

- diabetes during their lifetime.

MANAGING TYPE 2 DIABETES

Managing type 2 diabetes requires teamwork. You'll need to work closely with your doctor, but a lot of the results depend on your actions.

Your doctor may want to perform periodic blood tests to determine your blood sugar levels. This will help determine how well you're managing the disease. If you take medication, these tests will help gauge how well it's working.

Because diabetes increases your risk of cardiovascular disease, your doctor will also monitor your blood pressure and blood cholesterol levels. If you have symptoms of heart disease, you may need additional tests. These tests may include an electrocardiogram or a heart stress test.

Follow these tips to help manage your diabetes:

Maintain a diet high in nutrient-rich carbohydrates and fiber but low in unhealthy fats and simple carbohydrates.

Exercise daily.

- Take all your medication as recommended.

- Use a home monitoring system to test your blood sugar levels between visits to your doctor.

- Your doctor will tell you how often you should do that and what your target range should be.

It may also be helpful to bring your family into the loop. Educate them about the warning signs of blood sugar levels that are too high or too low so that they can help in an emergency. If everyone in your home follows a healthy diet and participates in physical activity, you'll all benefit.

Additional information on how to Managing Diabetes

You can manage your diabetes and live a long and healthy life by taking care of yourself each day. Diabetes can affect almost every part of your body. Therefore, you will need to manage your blood glucose levels, also called blood sugar. Managing your blood glucose, as well as your blood pressure and cholesterol, can help prevent the health problems that can occur when you have diabetes.

How can I manage my diabetes?

With the help of your health care team, you can create a diabetes self-care plan to manage your diabetes. Your self-care plan may include these steps:

- Manage your diabetes ABCs.

- Follow your diabetes meal plan.

- Make physical activity part of your routine.

- Take your medicine.

- Check your blood glucose levels.

- Work with your health care team.

- Cope with your diabetes in healthy ways.

- Manage your diabetes ABCs

Knowing your diabetes ABCs will help you manage your blood glucose, blood pressure, and cholesterol. Stopping smoking if you smoke will also help you manage your diabetes. Working toward your ABC goals can help lower your chances of having a heart attack, stroke, or other diabetes problems.

- A for the A1C test: The A1C test shows your average blood glucose level over the past 3 months. The A1C goal for many people with diabetes is below 7 percent. Ask your health care team what your goal should be.

- B for Blood pressure: The blood pressure goal for most people with diabetes is below 140/90 mm Hg. Ask what your goal should be.

- C for Cholesterol: You have two kinds of cholesterol in your blood: LDL and HDL. LDL or "bad" cholesterol can build up and clog your blood vessels. Too much bad cholesterol can cause a heart attack or stroke. HDL or "good" cholesterol helps remove the "bad" cholesterol from your blood vessels.

Ask your health care team what your cholesterol numbers should be. If you are over 40 years of age, you may need to take a statin drug for heart health.

- S for Stop smoking: Not smoking is especially important for people with diabetes because both smoking and diabetes narrow blood vessels. Blood vessel narrowing makes your heart work harder. E-cigarettes aren't a safe option either.

If you quit smoking you will lower your risk for heart attack, stroke, nerve disease, kidney disease, diabetic eye disease, and amputation. Your cholesterol and blood pressure levels may improve, your blood circulation will improve and you may have an easier time being physically active.

Keeping your A1C, blood pressure, and cholesterol levels close to your goals and stopping smoking may help prevent the long-term harmful effects of diabetes. These health problems include heart disease, stroke, kidney disease, nerve damage, and eye disease. You can keep track of your ABCs with a diabetes care record (568 KB). Take it with you on your health care visits. Talk about your goals and how you are doing, and whether you need to make any changes in your diabetes care plan.

• Follow your diabetes meal plan

Make a diabetes meal plan with help from your health care team. Following a meal plan will help you manage your blood glucose, blood pressure, and cholesterol.

Choose fruits and vegetables, beans, whole grains, chicken or turkey without the skin, fish, lean meats, and nonfat or low-fat milk and cheese. Drink water instead of sugar-sweetened beverages. Choose foods that are lower in calories, saturated fat, trans fat, sugar, and salt. Learn more about eating, diet, and nutrition with diabetes.

• Make physical activity part of your daily routine

Set a goal to be more physically active. Try to work up to 30 minutes or more of physical activity on most days of the week.

Brisk walking and swimming are good ways to move more. If you are not active now, ask your health care team about the types and amounts of physical activity that are right for you. Learn more about being physically active with diabetes.

Following your meal plan and being more active can help you stay at or get to a healthy weight. If you are overweight or obese, work with your health care team to create a weight-loss plan that is right for you.

- Take your medicine

Take your medicines for diabetes and any other health problems, even when you feel good or have reached your blood glucose, blood pressure, and cholesterol goals. These medicines help you manage your ABCs. Ask your doctor if you need to take aspirin to prevent a heart attack or stroke. Tell your health care professional if you cannot afford your medicines or if you have any side effects from your medicines. Learn more about insulin and other diabetes medicines.

- Check your blood glucose levels

For many people with diabetes, checking their blood glucose level each day is an important way to manage their diabetes. Monitoring your blood glucose level is most important if you take insulin. The results of blood glucose monitoring can help you make decisions about food, physical activity, and medicines.

- Checking and recording your blood glucose level is an important part of managing diabetes.

The most common way to check your blood glucose level at home is with a blood glucose meter. You get a drop of blood by pricking the side of your fingertip with a lancet. Then you apply the blood to a test strip. The meter will show you how much glucose is in your blood at the moment.

Ask your health care team how often you should check your blood glucose levels. Make sure to keep a record of your blood glucose self-checks. You can print copies of this glucose self-check chart (621 KB). Take these records with you when you visit your health care team.

What is continuous glucose monitoring?

Continuous glucose monitoring (CGM) is another way to check your glucose levels. Most CGM systems use a tiny sensor that you insert under your skin. The sensor measures glucose levels in the fluids between your body's cells every few minutes and can show changes in your glucose level throughout the day and night. If the CGM system shows that your glucose is too high or too low, you should check your glucose with a blood glucose meter before making any changes to your eating plan, physical activity, or medicines. A CGM system is especially useful for people who use insulin and have problems with low blood glucose.

What are the recommended targets for blood glucose levels?

Many people with diabetes aim to keep their blood glucose at these normal levels: Before a meal: 80 to 130 mg/dL About 2 hours after a meal starts: less than 180 mg/dL. Talk with your health care team about the best target range for you. Be sure to tell your health care professional if your glucose levels often go above or below your target range.

What happens if my blood glucose level becomes too low?

Sometimes blood glucose levels drop below where they should be, which is called hypoglycemia. For most people with diabetes, the blood glucose level is too low when it is below 70 mg/dL.Hypoglycemia can be life threatening and needs to be treated right away. Learn more about how to recognize and treat hypoglycemia.

What happens if my blood glucose level becomes too high?

Doctors call high blood glucose hyperglycemia.

Symptoms that your blood glucose levels may be too high include

- feeling thirsty

- feeling tired or weak

- headaches

- urinating often

- blurred vision

If you often have high blood glucose levels or symptoms of high blood glucose, talk with your health care team. You may need a change in your diabetes meal plan, physical activity plan, or medicines.

Know when to check for ketones

Your doctor may want you to check your urine for ketones if you have symptoms of diabetic ketoacidosis. When ketone levels get too high, you can develop this life-threatening condition.

Symptoms include

- trouble breathing

- nausea or vomiting

- pain in your abdomen

- Confusion

- feeling very tired or sleepy

Ketoacidosis most often is a problem for people with type 1 diabetes.

Work with your health care team. Most people with diabetes get health care from a primary care professional. Primary care professionals include internists, family physicians, and pediatricians. Sometimes physician assistants and nurses with extra training, called nurse practitioners, provide primary care. You also will need to see other care professionals from time to time. A team of health care professionals can help you improve your diabetes self-care. Remember, you are the most important member of your health care team.

Besides a primary care professional, your health care team may include an endocrinologist for more specialized diabetes care a registered dietitian, also called:

- a nutritionist

- a nurse

- a certified diabetes educator

- a pharmacist

- a dentist

- an eye doctor

- a podiatrist, or foot doctor, for foot care

- a social worker, who can help you find financial aid for treatment and community resources

- a counselor or other mental health care professional

When you see members of your health care team, ask questions. Write a list of questions you have before your visit so you don't forget what you want to ask. Watch a video to help you get ready for your diabetes care visit.

They are looking at a piece of paper. When you see your doctor, review your diabetes self-care plan and blood glucose chart. You should see your health care team at least twice a year, and more often if you are having problems or are having trouble reaching your blood glucose, blood pressure, or cholesterol goals. At each visit, be sure you have a blood pressure check, foot check, and weight check; and review your self-care plan. Talk with your health care team about your medicines and whether you need to adjust them. Routine health care will help you find and treat any health problems early, or may be able to help prevent them.

Talk with your doctor about what vaccines you should get to keep from getting sick, such as a flu shot and pneumonia shot. Preventing illness is an important part of taking care of your diabetes. Your blood glucose levels are more likely to go up when you're sick or have an infection. Learn more about taking care of your diabetes when you're sick and during other special times, such as when you're traveling.

• Cope with your diabetes in healthy ways

Feeling stressed, sad, or angry is common when you live with diabetes. Stress can raise your blood glucose levels, but you can learn ways to lower your stress. Try deep breathing, gardening, taking a walk, doing yoga, meditating, doing a hobby, or listening to your favorite music. Consider taking part in a diabetes education program or support group that teaches you techniques for managing stress. Learn more about healthy ways to cope with stress.

Depression is common among people with a chronic, or long-term, illness. Depression can get in the way of your efforts to manage your diabetes. Ask for help if you feel down. A mental health counselor, support group, clergy member, friend, or family member who will listen to your feelings may help you feel better.

Try to get 7 to 8 hours of sleep each night. Getting enough sleep can help improve your mood and energy level. You can take steps to improve your sleep habits. If you often feel sleepy during the day, you may have obstructive sleep apnea, a condition in which your breathing briefly stops many times during the night. Sleep apnea is common in people who have diabetes. Talk with your health care team if you think you have a sleep problem. Remember, managing diabetes isn't easy, but it's worth it

STEPS TO FIGHT DIABETES WITHOUT MEDICATION

Simple modification in lifestyle and some physical exercises daily can prevent pre-diabetic conditions.

Diabetes is a group of metabolic diseases in which the person has high blood glucose (blood sugar), either because insulin production is inadequate, or because the body's cells do not respond properly to insulin, or both.

Hypertension, gum disease, infections and stroke are some complications linked to badly controlled diabetes.

Simple modification in lifestyle and some physical exercises daily can prevent pre-diabetic conditions. Here are 10 ways to prevent diabetes:

1. Beans: Consumption of beans can help regulate blood glucose and insulin levels. They can help prevent diabetes, or minimize its effects in those diagnosed with the disease.

2. Almonds and walnuts: Almonds and walnuts prevent diabetes by regulating blood glucose. According to studies, eating almonds before a meal helps regulate blood sugar levels.

3. Green tea: As per studies, green tea regulates glucose levels in the body. It reduces complications associated with diabetes, such as cataract and cardiovascular disease, and promotes weight loss.

4. Blueberries: Consuming blueberries might help reduce the risk of diabetes, with the added benefit of helping you lose belly fat.

5. Exercise: At least 30 minutes of your day should be dedicated to exercise. It could be anything from walking to swimming. Regular exercise helps in reducing insulin resistance.

6. Adequate sleep: Get at least seven hours of sleep daily. A University of Chicago study found that people who slept for less than six hours each night were at a higher risk of diabetes.

7. Fish: Eat fish once a week. Docosahexaenoic acid (DHA) and eicosapentaenoic acid (EPA) can help improve insulin sensitivity.

8. Sunshine: Get enough of sunshine vitamin. Scientists say that the people with high levels of vitamin D are less likely to develop type II diabetes.

9. Citrus fruits: Oranges, grapefruit and other citrus fruits are rich in vitamin C, which helps keep the heart healthy. Opt for whole fruit. Fiber in whole fruit slows sugar absorption so you get the citrus fruit nutrients without sending your blood sugar soaring.

10. Whole grains. Pearled barley, oatmeal, breads and other whole-grain foods are high in fiber and contain nutrients such as magnesium, chromium, folate and omega 3 fatty acids.

THE SAFEST FIRST-LINE THERAPY FOR TYPE 2 DIABETES

According to more than 200 studies involving 1.4 million patients, metformin reduces heart disease risk in diabetes patients more effectively than its competitors.

A recent meta-analysis, published in the Annals of Internal Medicine, found metformin, widely used for treating type 2 diabetes (T2D), was safer for the heart than many newer competitors. Metformin showed particularly dramatic results when compared to sulfonylurea, its closest competitor drug, reducing the relative risk of a patient dying from heart disease by about 30 – 40 percent.

Paired reviewers independently identified 179 trials and 25 observational studies of head-to-head monotherapy or metformin-based combinations. And two reviewers independently assessed study quality and serially extracted data and graded the strength of evidence. The results showed that cardiovascular mortality was lower for metformin versus sulfonylureas; the evidence on all-cause mortality, cardiovascular morbidity, and microvascular complications was insufficient or of low strength. Reductions in hemoglobin A1C values were similar across monotherapies and metformin-based combinations, except that DPP-4 inhibitors had smaller effects. Body weight was reduced or maintained with metformin, DPP-4 inhibitors, GLP-1 receptor agonists, and SGLT-2 inhibitors and increased with sulfonylureas, thiazolidinediones, and insulin (between-group differences up to 5 kg). Hypoglycemia was more frequent with sulfonylureas. Gastrointestinal adverse events were highest with metformin and GLP-1 receptor agonists. Genital mycotic infections were increased with SGLT-2 inhibitors.

From the results it was concluded that the evidence supports metformin again as the first-line therapy for type 2 diabetes, given its relative safety and beneficial effects on hemoglobin A1c, weight, and cardiovascular mortality (compared with sulfonylureas). Added to the conclusions was that metformin is the only antidiabetic agent that has shown reduced macrovascular outcomes, which is likely explained by its effects beyond glycemic control. It has also been employed as an adjunct to lifestyle modifications in prediabetes and insulin-resistant states. A large amount of evidence in literature supports its use even in cases where it would be contra-indicated mainly due to the fear of lactic acidosis, which has been over-emphasized as the available data suggest that lactate levels and risk of lactic acidosis do not differ appreciably in patients taking this drug versus other glucose-lowering agents. It has also recently gained attention as potential treatment for neurodegenerative diseases such as Alzheimer's disease.

Metformin acts primarily at the liver by reducing glucose output and, secondarily, by augmenting glucose uptake in the peripheral tissues, chiefly muscle. These effects are mediated by the activation of an upstream kinase, liver kinase B1 (LKB-1), which in turn regulates the downstream kinase adenosine monophosphatase protein kinase (AMPK). AMPK phosphorylates a transcriptional co-activator, transducer of regulated CREB protein 2 (TORC2), resulting in its inactivation, which consequently downregulates transcriptional events that promote synthesis of gluconeogenic enzymes. Inhibition of mitochondrial respiration has also been proposed to contribute to the reduction of gluconeogenesis since it reduces the energy supply required for this process.

Metformin's efficacy, security profile, benefic cardiovascular and metabolic effects, and its capacity to be associated with other antidiabetic agents makes this drug the first glucose lowering agent of choice when treating patients with type 2 diabetes mellitus (TDM2).

Several other classes of oral antidiabetic agents have been recently launched, introducing the need to evaluate the role of metformin as initial therapy and in combination with this newer drugs. There is increasing evidence from in vivo and in vitro studies supporting its anti-proliferative role in cancer and possibly a neuroprotective effect. Metformin's negligible risk of hypoglycemia in monotherapy and few drug interactions of clinical relevance give this drug a high safety profile. The tolerability of metformin may be improved by using an appropriate dose titration, starting with low doses, so that side-effects can be minimized or by switching to an extended release form.

Practice Pearls:

Metformin acts primarily at the liver by reducing glucose output and, secondarily, by augmenting glucose uptake in the peripheral tissues, chiefly muscle.

The first glucose-lowering agent of choice when treating patients with type 2 diabetes mellitus (TDM2).

Metformin is the only antidiabetic agent that has shown reduced macrovascular outcomes which is likely explained by its effects beyond glycemic control.

EXERCISE TIPS FOR TYPE 2 DIABETES

Exercise is sure to be on your to-do list if you have diabetes. Get started with these go-to tips:

1. Make a list of fun activities. You have lots of options, and you don't have to go to a gym. What sounds good? Think about something you've always wanted to try or something you enjoyed in the past. Sports, dancing, yoga, walking, and swimming are a few ideas. Anything that raises your heart rate counts.

2. Get your doctor's OK. Let them know what you want to do. They can make sure you're ready for it. They'll also check to see if you need to change your meals, insulin, or diabetes medicines. Your doctor can also let you know if the time of day you exercise matters.

3. Check your blood sugar. Ask your doctor if you should check it before exercise. If you plan to work out for more than an hour, check your blood sugar levels regularly during your workout, so you'll know if you need a snack. Check your blood sugar after every workout, so that you can adjust if needed.

4. Carry carbs. Always keep a small carbohydrate snack, like fruit or a fruit drink, on hand in case your blood sugar gets low.

5. Ease into it. If you're not active now, start with 10 minutes of exercise at a time. Gradually work up to 30 minutes a day.

6. Strength train at least twice a week. It can improve blood sugar control. You can lift weights or work with resistance bands. Or you can do moves like push-ups, lunges, and squats, which use your own body weight.

7. Make it a habit. Exercise, eat, and take your medicines at the same time each day to prevent low blood sugar, also called hypoglycemia.

8. Go public. Work out with someone who knows you have diabetes and knows what to do if your blood sugar gets too low. It's more fun, too. Also wear a medical identification tag, or carry a card that says you have diabetes, just in case.

9. Be good to your feet. Wear athletic shoes that are in good shape and are the right type for your activity. For instance, don't jog in tennis shoes, because your foot needs a different type of support when you run. Check and clean your feet daily. Let your doctor know if you notice any new foot problems.

10. Hydrate. Drink water before, during, and after exercise.

11. Stop if something suddenly hurts. If your muscles are mildly sore, that's normal. Sudden pain isn't. You're not likely to get injured unless you do too much, too soon.

Health Benefits You'll Get

Remember how much exercise does for you, including:

i. Helps your body use insulin, which controls your blood sugar

ii. Burns extra body fat

iii. Strengthens muscles and bones

iv. Lowers blood pressure

v. Cuts LDL ("bad") cholesterol

vi. Raises HDL ("good") cholesterol

vii. Improves blood flow

viii. Makes heart disease and stroke less likely

ix. Boosts energy and mood

x. Tames stress

THE IMPORTANCE OF EXERCISE IN FIGHTING TYPE 2 DIABETES

As more and more of us are leading less active lives and, for example, sitting all day long in our ergonomic chairs in front of a computer, health problems associated with this change in our lifestyle are rising.

I don't think that anybody would dispute the fact we need to take some regular exercise, but only about 30% of people in the United States are currently getting the recommended level of thirty minutes exercise a day and it is frightening to discover that 25% of Americans today take very little or no exercise at all.

So what does this have to do with type 2 diabetes?

In recent years, in large part as a result of lower levels of activity, we have seen a dramatic increase in the number of people who are overweight in the United States and indeed obesity in America has now reached epidemic proportions. One major side-effect of this is that, as weight rises, so does insulin resistance and the onset of type 2 diabetes.

If you are skeptical about the connection between weight and diabetes then you only need to look at the latest statistics from the US Department of Health and Human Services which show that a staggering 80% of people suffering from type 2 diabetes are also classed as being clinically overweight.

If we are to reverse the rising trend in the number of people being diagnosed with type 2 diabetes then we must attack one of its root causes which is increasing weight. In turn, this means looking carefully at our diet but, just as importantly, looking at the amount of exercise we take to burn off the calories we are eating.

Perhaps the biggest problem whenever anyone mentions exercise is that it conjures up a picture of having to put on a pair of sweat pants and a tee shirt and jog around the local park or join those fitness fanatics down at the local gym. Nothing could be farther from the truth. Of course, you can go jogging if you want to, or join your local gym, but there are numerous other options open to you.

The secret is simply to add activity into your daily routine which stretches you physically. Not to the point at which you feel you are about to collapse, but simply to the point at which you are aware of making your body do a bit of extra work.

So what sort of things are we talking about?

Well, if you live in an apartment on the fifth floor, use the stairs instead of taking the lift. If you ride the bus to work, get off a couple of stops early and walk the last part of your journey. If your garden is in need of attention, get out once or twice a week and push the mower around, do some weeding or dig over the vegetable patch.

This list of exercise opportunities is virtually endless and it doesn't really matter how you get your exercise. What is important is that you look carefully at your lifestyle and, in particular, at your daily routine and try to work in at least 30 minutes of physical activity every day. Combine this with taking a close look at your eating habits and both your weight and the problems associated with type 2 diabetes will begin to fall.

HOW TO FIGHT DIABETES EFFECTIVELY

With diabetes reaching epidemic levels, it is important to understand how to fight diabetes. Thankfully, it is not always as challenging as many people think.

There are 2 big things that you need to keep in mind if you want to know how to fight diabetes. These are exercise and nutrition.

How To Fight Diabetes With Nutrition

What you eat can help prevent, or even reverse diabetes. The key is to focus on high nutrient, low-calorie foods. It is important to understand what the glycemic index (GI) is. Simply put, the GI rates foods based on how they affect your blood sugar. The lower the score, the better job the food does keeping your blood sugar levels steady. This is important for a few reasons. First, it prevents the "sugar highs" and crashes. Second, it helps keep you feeling full longer. Also, it helps prevent cravings, along with keeping a steady mood throughout the day. In the fight against diabetes, the glycemic index is an important tool.

Foods with a score of 55 or less are considered beneficial to your health. These foods are typically vegetables, and some fruits. Focus on whole grain products instead of white, heavily processed ones. Stay away from soda, and drink plenty of water. Regardless of what some diets may tell you, do not eliminate protein, carbs or fat from your diet. All 3 of those are essential to proper body function. Restricting your nutrient intake is not a healthy way to lose weight, nor is it how to fight diabetes. Think before you eat, and focus on a healthy balance of fruits, vegetables, whole grains and healthy fats, such as in chicken or fish.

How To Fight Diabetes With Exercises

Exercise is another powerful tool in the fight against diabetes. When you exercises, you are doing a few different things to your body. First, you are burning calories, and in effect, melting away fat. Second, your metabolism kicks into gear, which helps your body process everything more effectively. As you get in better shape, your body can become more sensitive to insulin, which is very important if you are trying to prevent or reverse diabetes. It is important that when you start exercising, you understand some basic rules.

- Make sure that you know your limits. Pushing too hard right away can lead to a lot of complications that will only set you back.

- Stay hydrated - When you are working out, sip water throughout the workout. If you become dehydrated, you may end up doing harm to your body.

- Mix in strength, cardio and flexibility training for maximum results.

MASSAGE THERAPY FOR DIABETES

Massage therapy can often help in relieving symptoms of diabetes. If you or a loved one suffers from this life-altering disease, you are familiar with the time and effort it takes to regain and maintain a healthy lifestyle. Apart from injections, continual monitoring and dietary changes, what can diabetes patients do to reduce stress and promote longevity?

The Physical and Emotional Damage of Diabetes

Diabetes affects the body's ability to either produce or use insulin, the naturally occurring hormone that assists in transferring glucose to the body's cells. In both Type 1 and Type 2 diabetes, blood glucose levels are raised, starving the patient's body of energy. The most immediate physical reaction is fatigue, but extremely high blood glucose levels become dangerous, especially when the body is subjected to them over periods of time. Cell damage begins to occur in the kidneys, heart, eyes and other organs. Once diagnosed with diabetes, patients must keep a permanent watchful eye on their condition in order to preserve their health.

Diabetes is not only a disease affecting the body. Daily injections, constant blood glucose level checks, and the need for regular check-ins with physicians can take an emotional toll as well. Diabetes patients are twice as likely to encounter depression, according to data collected by the National Institute for Mental Health. With one out of every 10 adults over age 20 suffering from diabetes, it's important to exhaust each and every treatment option in the hopes of maintaining equilibrium in body and mind, and massage therapy offers specific benefits for diabetes patients.

Benefits of Regular Massages

The main obstacle facing diabetes patients is insulin absorption. Since many patients have poor circulation, massage is an ideal solution, as it stimulates the lymph system, encouraging the cells to improve insulin absorption function.

A common side effect of diabetes is stiff or inflamed joints. When glucose levels are high, the connective tissues and muscles suffer a lack of mobility or lowered range of motion. Massage works against a thickened myofascial system and improves litheness of the muscles.

According to the American Massage Therapy Association, after only a 15-minute chair massage, studied subjects all showed significantly lower levels of stress and improvements in their emotional state. For diabetic patients living with daily challenges, reducing anxiety is a major hurdle to overcome on their path to lifelong wellness.

Potential Risks

After a massage, patients might feel light-headed or disoriented. It is vitally important for diabetic massage therapy patients to test their blood sugar levels and ensure they are not suffering from low blood sugar. This state, also called hypoglycemia, includes feeling dizzy and fatigued.

Additionally, diabetic patients must inform their practitioner of their condition and take note of how their blood sugar levels respond to a massage. Each individual reaction is different, but glucose levels typically drop between 20 and 40 milligrams per deciliter.

Form a safe, personalized trial treatment plan after consulting with your physician before utilizing massage therapy or a massage chair. Expect to see massage therapy help diabetes symptoms recede due to physical relaxation, leading to emotional and mental well-being.

www.ingramcontent.com/pod-product-compliance
Lightning Source LLC
Chambersburg PA
CBHW070103210526
45170CB00012B/733